by Dan Fielder

Illustrations by Neil Bennett

Cover by Jim Lefevre

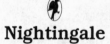

Nightingale

An imprint of Wimbledon Publishing Company
LONDON

Copyright © 2000
Illustrations © 2000 WPC

First published in Great Britain in 2000
by Wimbledon Publishing Company Ltd
P.O. Box 9779 London SW19 7ZG
All rights reserved

First published 2000 in Great Britain

ISBN: 1903222 15 X

Produced in Great Britain
Printed and bound in Hungary

There is at least one world record that all of us - right now - are trying to break. That record is the one for longevity. Currently the official holder is one Jeanne Calmant, a French woman who died in 1997 at the age of 122 years and 153 days.

We can all learn a lot from Mme Calmant, who knew Van Gogh, enjoyed a glass of port each day, ate Swiss chocolate and only gave up smoking at 110 on the grounds that 'it was becoming a habit'. Such 'centenarians' are frequently eccentric, stubborn and outspoken people.

But they are also independent, resourceful and fiercely loyal - to themselves, their friends and families, and their beliefs. This little collection of tips and thoughts attempts to uncover something of their secret, and is dedicated to their tenacious love of life.

Dan Fielder
1999

BODY

Cold start

Start the day with a warm shower followed by a two-minute blast of cold water. According to recent British research, cold showers can make your heart and lungs work efficiently, boost immunity and reduce the risk of heart attacks.

'Be positive and optimistic. Believe in yourself. Smile a lot. Never smoke. Drink very moderately. Take aerobic exercise three times a week. Take an 81mg (baby) aspirin every night before bed. Achieve peace of mind around you...and you'll hit 100.'

Uri Geller

Healthy eating = long life

Eating fresh fruit and veg gives you a better chance of dying in your bed. A study of 3000 Finnish, Dutch and Italian people found that those whose diets were most in line with World Health Organisation guidelines - which recommend five portions of fresh produce every day - cut their risk of dying an untimely death by 13%.

(British Medical Journal)

'I've lived this long because I refused to die! I have good friends, I'm healthy. Above all, I'm active.'
Dirk Struik, mathematics professor, 104

Kick the weed!

If you smoke, giving up is the single biggest thing you can do to boost your health and prolong your life. Smoking-related illnesses such as lung cancer and emphysema are major causes of death in the UK - accounting for 120,000 deaths every single year.

Go nuts

It's time to open your life to more raw, unsalted nuts. An extensive survey of women's health found that a diet including 150g (5oz) of nuts per week reduces your risk of heart attack (as compared to those who never eat nuts) by one-third. Go for almonds, walnuts and peanuts.

Keeping it in the family

Having a very old sibling increases your own survival chances. Brothers and sisters of people who live to be 100 are four times as likely to live into their nineties themselves than siblings of people born in the same era who died in their early Seventies.

Supplementary benefits

The main cause of ageing is oxidation, caused by particles known as free radicals which stress and damage the body. The key to longevity is to neutralise free radical damage by increasing your intake of antioxidant nutrients such as vitamin A, C, E, selenium, zinc, glutathione and flavonoids.

'Cut back on your intake of oxidants from smoking, fried foods and pollution. My key daily supplement would be a good multivitamin plus an antioxidant complex, giving optimum amounts of these nutrients. This strategy is likely to add 15 years to your life - and life to your years!'

Patrick Holford, founder of the Institute of Optimum Nutrition

Sing up

Whether it's in the shower or down at the karaoke night, a good sing-song can work wonders. It helps you express yourself, reducing the likelihood of depressive thoughts, and it's also surprisingly aerobic - giving your inner organs a real workout.

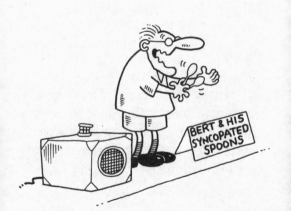

Hop, skip or jump

Starting the day by jumping or skipping on the spot 50 times can prolong you life, a study at Nottingham University found. The exercise helps strengthen the heart, guard against cardiovascular disease, and reduce the risk of osteoporosis.

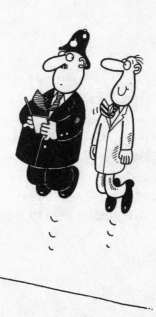

Breathing space

When things are getting on top of you, pause for a moment. Breathe in through your nose for a count of four, and out through your mouth for five. Relax the shoulders, and repeat.

'*Only about 30 per cent of the characteristics of ageing are genetically determined. The other 70 per cent are linked to lifestyle.*'

James Rowe, gerontologist

'I always go to bed early, and rarely go out in the evening. I still teach music part-time, but always finish by 5.30pm. After a meal I am usually in bed by 6.30pm, with my radio, tapes, television and books. - I love it! I rarely sleep before midnight, I only need five hours or so sleep.'

Anna Hewitt, 85

Eat pumpkin seeds

They contain a substance called tryptophan, which can help raise levels of the mood-enhancing brain chemical serotonin.

Work that body!

For a noticeable improvement in life expectancy, according to Dr Ronald Klatz of the American Academy of Anti-Ageing Medicine, you need to do at least 20 minutes of continuous aerobic exercise three times a week, coupled with 30 minutes of daily exercise such as gardening or housework.

Club Med

Nutritionists agree that for a life-long healthy eating plan, we could all benefit from following the example of the Mediterranean countries. The southern European diet includes pasta, lots of fresh fruit and veg, salads, garlic and olive oil. Some experts see olive oil as the real secret of longevity - it contains vitamin E, which helps keep arteries unblocked, and monounsaturated fats, which lowers blood cholesterol and reduces the risk of atherosclerosis.

Know your body

Make an appointment to see your GP if you come across any of the following symptoms, which may be linked with an illness in need of treatment: a noticeable and sudden change in weight; unexplained pain or bleeding; swelling or lumps; a sore which doesn't heal; changes to a mole or wart; indigestion or problems with swallowing for more than two weeks; persistent hoarseness or coughing; changes in bowel or bladder habits that last over two weeks.

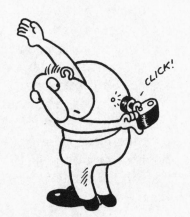

Be a woman!

Statistically women have long outlived men. The life expectancy for a man born between 1985 and 1990 is 72.4 years; a woman can expect to live an average 78.1 years. One reason for this is that women are naturally better protected from heart disease - at least until the menopause - by the female hormone oestrogen. In 1990, America had 37,306 centenarians - 29,405 of them women.

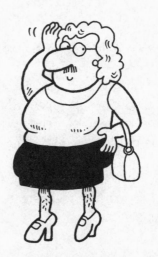

...or talk to one

Men gain more reassurance from talking to women than to men. In University of California tests on male blood pressure, men with a wife or several female friends were found to be much more likely to cope with the type of stress linked with heart disease. All of which adds weight to the theory that married men are healthier than single ones.

Eat more fish

Fish contains essential B vitamins for brain power and essential fatty acids to protect against heart disease. Edible bones in oily fish provide calcium to protect against osteoporosis.

Develop good sleeping habits

The importance of sleep to our health is much underrated. Regular and sufficient slumber improves memory, repairs the body better, and boosts immunity to illness, mood and coping skills. Aim to be in bed by midnight, and to develop a regular sleeping pattern.

Cut out salt

Cutting your salt intake by half (from 10g to 5g per day) can help you lose weight even without dieting. It's worth the sacrifice - lower salt levels help lower blood pressure, reduce the risk of stroke, prevent osteoporosis and reduce asthma attacks.

'Golf teaches you so many lessons in life. It teaches you not to get cocky. It teaches you to be punctual. if the world could be run like golf, there would be no murders, rapes and drugs.'

Gary Player, still playing top-flight golf at 64

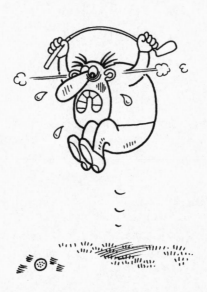

Prevention is better than cure

Cardiovascular disease is one of the biggest causes of premature death in Britain, accounting for 300,000 lives every year. A healthy diet and regular exercise offer protection. Natural heart boosters include garlic, onion, ginger and folic acid, which is found in green leafy veg, broccoli, sprouts, pulses, wheat germ, fortified cereal and bread. Recent research links folic acid with reduced blood levels of homocysteine, thought to be a major risk factor.

If it hurts, it won't last

Keeping active is essential to a long life, but there's no point going to the gym or taking up running if you can't stand those activities. Whether it's tennis or dancing, find a form or exercise you love, and join a club: paying money up front is extra motivation.

Long-life breakfast

Breakfast is the most important meal of the day, helping to kickstart the metabolism and rehydrate the body. Make up your first meal of the day from the following options: eggs and wholemeal bread; a bowl of oats; fruit - a peach, mango or orange; a low-fat yoghurt.

The hormone factor

Anti-ageing researchers are looking more and more to 'super-hormones' in the fight to look and feel younger. One popular supplement is DHEA, a hormone produced by the adrenal glands in levels that peak at the age of 25 and decline rapidly thereafter. Its supporters say that if you maintain DHEA at peak levels, you can actually wind back your internal 'ageing clock' so that your cells still believe they're in their twenties - long after you're not!

Youthful yoga

Yoga is suitable for people of all ages and abilities, and can help slow down the ageing process. 'Yoga has a rejuvenating effect on mind and body, not only of maintaining a fit and toned body but also by regulating the metabolism, balancing the hormone system and raising energy levels,' says teacher Vimla Lalvani.

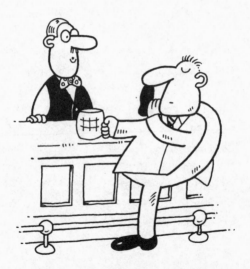

Don't be a slob

There's no escaping it: people with unhealthy lifestyles pay for it later. A survey of 1,741 former students of the University of Pennsylvania found that the people who smoked, were overweight and didn't exercise enough had twice as much disability as those who'd lived more healthily and who enjoyed, on average, an extra five years of fitness.

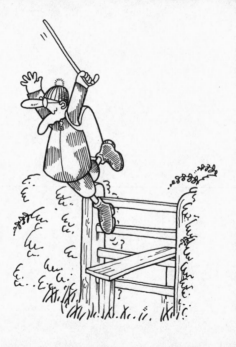

From here to maternity

Women who have a child in their 40s are four times more likely to die at 100 than at 73.

Avoid lie-ins

Staying in bed all morning at the weekend is not the tonic you might think. Sleep researchers have found that sleeping in can actually lead to feelings of incompetence and irritability - symptoms similar to those associated with sleep deprivation.

Chocolate: just say yes

Here's a tough tip - eat chocolate and live longer! A survey of 8000 Harvard graduates showed that those who ate one to three chocolate bars a month enjoyed greater longevity. The highest mortality rate fell to the group who ate no chocolate at all.

Have a green cuppa

According to Japanese research, green tea improves longevity and reduces the risk of lung cancer and stroke. Normal tea, too, is thought to lower blood cholesterol and blood pressure.

Go organic

Pollutants such as pesticides and lead are thought to adversely affect the working of the immune system. Organic produce - from supermarkets to box-delivery schemes - is increasingly available. Or wash fruit and veg in a solution of warm water and vinegar for five minutes to help remove any potentially harmful residues.

'Choose your genes; eat your beans
Take a tot; walk a lot.
Though snappy, make someone happy.
Avoid fret, get a pet
And use your brain or it will wane.'
Dr Michael Apple, GP and author

Touchy-feely

'For a long and healthy life you ought to have massage - and give massage too,' says therapist Clare Maxwell-Hudson. 'In a study of volunteer grandparents in Miami, giving a massage actually made people feel better than receiving one. It gives you *joie de vivre* - and helps keep you active.'

'I get up every day with a positive attitude because I have always got jobs and activities planned, whether in the home or the voluntary community work I've always been involved in. And walking everywhere keeps me fit.'

Rose Ball, 85

It's never too late to work out

Muscle weakening may not be an inevitable side effect of growing old. Researchers in Massachusetts found that 80 and 90-year-olds given weight-lifting exercises significantly increased muscle size and strength after just eight weeks. The training helped them become more mobile, and less dependent on canes and even wheelchairs.

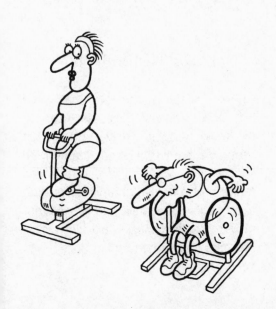

Snack healthily

Many nutritionists believe that 'little but often' is the best way to eat healthily. Regular, smaller intakes of food will help to prevent your blood sugar levels from falling, which can make you more vulnerable to disease and have a negative effect on your mood. Healthy snacks include raisins, oat bars and sugar-free liquorice.

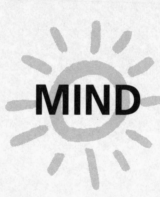

Manage stress effectively

Stress is the plague of our century and a major obstacle to long life. Although stress-related problems are often experienced as something in the mind, the effects on the body are all too real: high blood pressure, depleted immunity, poor digestion, migraine, IBS, asthma, eczema, heart disease... Useful stressbusters include taking regular breaks, learning to say no, and correcting your posture at work.

Do something you enjoy - now!

It's official: happiness makes you healthy. Pleasant experiences stimulate the release of protective antibodies such as immunoglobin-A. So whether it's eating out or reading a good book, you owe it to yourself to have a good time at once...

'Eat the right food, exercise, and remain mentally curious.'

Eli Finn, 102

Wear odd socks

Daring to be different can be a powerful medicine. A wide-ranging study of eccentric people found them to be highly creative, energetic and optimistic. They live longer than average, and visit the doctor far less. It is thought that they do better because they see no need to conform, and refuse to acknowledge failure, so feel little of the stress that can be so damaging the body's immune system.

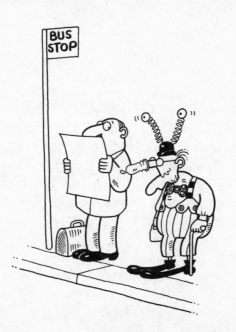

Do your paperwork early

Research into circadian rhythms - the body's internal clock - shows that we are best prepared for intellectual and mental work between 7am and midday.

Have a laugh

Laughter deepens the breath, boosts immunity and triggers the release of the body's own painkiller and feel-good drugs. In his book *Anatomy of an Illness*, Norman Cousins explains how he recovered from an apparently incurable illness by reading funny books and watching Marx Brothers videos to keep himself in a constant good mood.

Healthy and wealthy

American and European research repeatedly shows a direct link between income and health. In one study of 300,000 American men, there were significant improvements in health for every US$2000 you went up the income scale. A man on US$26,000, for instance, lives noticeably longer than a man on US$24,000.

Congratulations!

Make a point of rewarding yourself whenever you finish a laborious or dreaded task. Even if it's just buying a favourite magazine or calling a friend, it pays to appreciate your own efforts.

Clean up your thoughts

Develop a healthier attitude by getting rid of all your negative and unhelpful thought patterns. Avoid phrases like 'I can't' or 'I'm hopeless'. Replace with something like 'I'll do my best' or 'I'm getting better at...'. Turn 'problems' into 'challenges' and 'nervousness' into 'excitement'. Avoid words like 'ought', 'should', 'fault' and 'blame'.

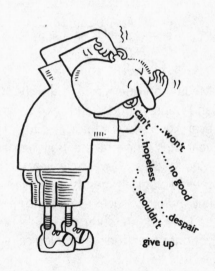

Don't medicate - meditate!

Meditation doesn't just calm the mind and improve focus and mood - it can even keep you youthful. A study of 50-year olds who practise Transcendental Meditation for over five years found their biological age (as determined by key markers such as hearing, vision and blood pressure) to be 12 years younger than their chronological age.

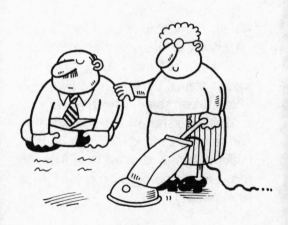

Embrace a trunk

A native American custom for warding off illness involves going into the forest and sitting with your back against a mature tree. If that sounds a bit much, at least keep some greenery near you: studies have shown that time spent in nature boosts mood, and that hospital patients with a view of trees tend to recover more quickly than those cut off from nature.

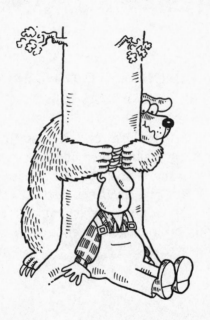

Don't give up the crossword...

A survey of 100 centenarians found that what all of them had in common was some regular form of intellectual activity. 'The mind has resources that can be called on when the frailty of the body takes over,' concluded researchers.

Not now…

One American study of very old people ran into an unexpected difficulty. Several people over 100 refused to participate - on the grounds that they were too busy.

Eastern promise

Adopting a daily practice such as *t'ai chi* can reap dividends. Research by the US National Institute on Ageing found that practising *t'ai chi* three times a week improved balance and helped prevent falls in the elderly. It has also been associated with reducing stress and blood pressure, and improving circulation, heart and hormonal function.

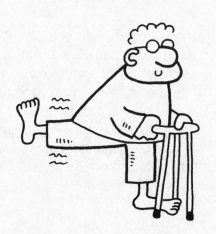

Have a good cry

Having a good blub when the mood takes you is something not nearly enough of us do - only one in eight people admit to crying frequently, according to a recent survey. But tears are a good thing, removing chemicals from the body that are built up during stress - which is why, after the release, you always feel better.

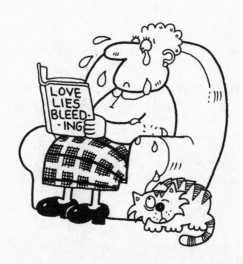

Animal attraction

Whether it's a llama or a goldfish, a pet is a great tonic. Companion animals have been found to give comfort to their owners in times of trouble and to reduce the blood pressure of people under moderate stress. Even watching ornamental fish has a proven relaxing effect.

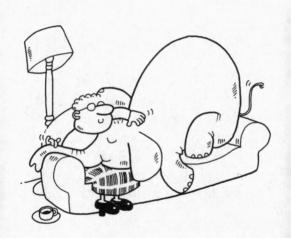

Leave the office on time

Long working hours can raise stress levels, and lead to headaches, repetitive strain injury and heart disease. Four million people in the UK now work more than 48 hours a week - the highest rate in Europe - and the health risks rise with every extra hour.

Instant stressbuster

If you feel tensions soaring, take a few minutes out from what you are doing. Starting at your feet, slowly relax every muscle of your body, ending with your facial muscles. If you don't have the time, simple close your eyes and clench and unclench your fists.

Be yourself,
warts and all

A University of Georgia study of people 100 years old and over found no 'secret formula' to a long life - except, possibly state of mind. Many of the centenarians had smoked, drunk heavily, or worked for years out in the sun, and been brought up on diets of bacon, butter and full-fat milk. But they were also found to be more stubborn, more aggressive and more suspicious than their younger counterparts.

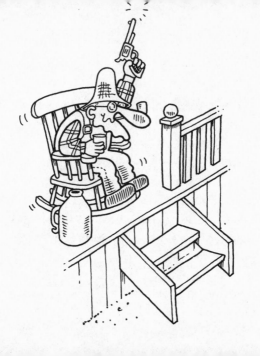

'Keep yourself as busy as possible - doing what you like best. Don't do as other people suggest. Follow your own instincts.'

Jack Thain, General-Secretary, National Pensioners' Convention. At 77, he still works an unpaid seven-day week

Learn to relax

Real relaxation is a powerful stress-buster. A soak in a bath with essential oils or listening to a self-hypnosis tape can work wonders.

Lay off the Scratchcards

For a long and contented life, a non-materialistic attitude could be crucial. According to US psychologist Cecilia Hurwich, realising that money doesn't buy happiness will give you greater optimism - a key factor in longevity. Also, bear in mind that, statistically, the very rich have an above-average probability of dying young...

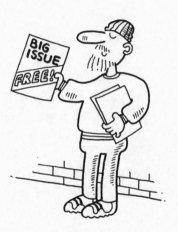

Save the tough stuff for Tuesdays!

Research suggests that Tuesday is the day of the working week when we are most alert and perfom best. On Mondays we're still out of sync from the weekend, and by Wednesday we're already getting tired…

Keep something back

Make a list of five instant feel-good factors - things that you know will instantly put you in a good mood. Dip into this reserve of quick fixes whenever you experience a sudden low.

What's yours?

Sharing a joke at the pub can keep you in clover for longer. Psychologists at the University of Hull found that, of 322 social drinkers, those who drank more were less stressed and had a greater propensity to see the funny side of life.

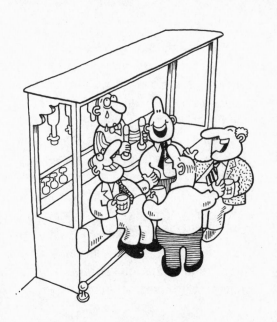

From verse to better...

Reading and writing poetry can be a therapy in itself. Research at Bristol University found that people who read verse were able to improve stress and brighten their frame of mind. Those who penned poems themselves, meanwhile, benefited from a powerful emotional outlet. 'It seems that the rhythm and subject of poetry can have a reassuring and calming effect, in part by demonstrating that others have felt the same as you,' commented one expert.

Award yourself a 'duvet day'!

If you're feeling down or anxious, dragging yourself into the office can make you feel worse. Call in sick - and don't allow yourself to feel guilty about it.

Keep talking

Phoning a friend for a chat is good for you. People who enjoy a diverse social life have been found to be less likely to catch colds than those who had regular contact with fewer than five people.

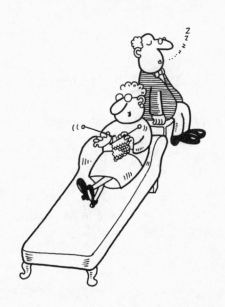

A look at bedtime

Improve your memory and enrich your experience by spending a few minutes going through the day in your mind before you go to sleep. Try to remember snatches of specific conversations, TV theme tunes, the clothes people were wearing.

SPIRIT

Go to church

American researchers found that people who regularly attend services have a longer life expectancy than those who dton't - not least because they benefit from a wider 'support network' of friends.

Olé!

The Spanish word for a retired person is 'jubilado' - as in jubilant!

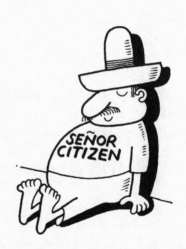

'As often as possible, I try to remember to say the following "Forgiveness Prayer":

'I declare today a day of amnesty in which I gratefully volunteer to hand in all of my resentments and grievances to You. Please help me to handle well all of the peace that must inevitably follow."

Robert Holden, founder of the first NHS Laughter Clinic

Think alternative

From aromatherapy to shiatsu, complementary therapies can help with many of the stress-related problems that are so common today. And by focusing on the underlying causes of illness in your lifestyle, they can help keep them at bay too.

An attitude of gratitude

Get into the habit of looking at your life in terms of what you already have - rather than beating yourself up for what's missing. An easy way to do this is to write or recite a thank-you list of all the things in your life - people, experiences, situations, objects - that you wouldn't want to be without.

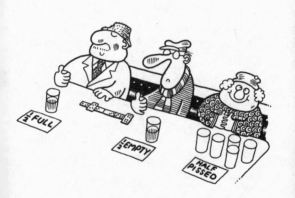

'The great secret that all old people share is that you really haven't changed in 70 or 80 years; your body changes but you haven't changed at all.'

Doris Lessing

'The older you get, the older you want to get.'

Keith Richards

Forthcoming title

At the age of 105, Mary Sims Elliott published her autobiography. She called it *My First One Hundred Years*.

Think abundantly

Don't let money worries stress you out. See money as an energy, which flows in and out of our lives. The more you encourage the flow - through unconditional giving, for instance - the more you'll get back. Adopt the attitude that there really is more than enough to go round.

Get it off your chest

Emotional honesty can have an impact on health. In University of Miami research, students were asked to discuss stressful and traumatic events. Those who revealed the most were also found to have the best immune system.

Don't give up the day job...

Groups of people who live longer than average include business leaders who don't retire, orchestra conductors, successful artists, women listed in *Who's Who*, and Mormons. Being active and dedicated to your occupation - whatever the stresses - is clearly less harmful than the monotony that can come with being under-occupied.

'Old age isn't so bad when you consider the alternatives.'

Maurice Chevalier

'Keep on raging - to stop the ageing'
The Delltones

'Today's long-livers are generally happier with much less - they had much lower expectations than younger generations today. They usually walked alot, had more physical lives, and slept better. People seem to live longer in tight-knit communities with extended families nearby, where they know people care about them - many lonely or isolated people give up on life. Today's elderly are not so knocked sideways by traumatic events because they became mentally strong through experiencing a World War (or two).'

Mary Forsyth, community nurse

'It is not how old you are, but how you are old.'

Marie Dressler

Till death do us part…

Not surprisingly, a long, happy marriage equals a long, happy life. In a Florida study of 69 people over 100, some 50 had been married for over 30 years - and two for over 70 years!

'I have learned that I can earn a living doing what I love, which both gives me joy and helps other people. I have realised that it is arrogant to put ourselves down - our creator loves us without conditions. Our only real job is to love ourselves and each other.'

Nick Williams, author of
The Work We Were Born To

'The secret of a long and happy existence is to keep yourself rooted in your family and friends - don't let ambition take over your life.'
Cary Cooper, stress management guru

'I had always nursed a secret ambition to paint and write and, after my husband died when I was 78, I entered a real creative period. I did a writing course and learned to use a computer. Now I travel when I can afford to, and write and paint constantly. And my daily early morning spiritual reading helps me to focus on a target for the day.'

Mary Hunt, 85

Work at love

Couples who think they met by fate and then argue a lot have been found to suffer more depression than couples who believe relationships require time and effort to develop.

'Know yourself, be yourself, enjoy yourself - and avoid living up to other people's expectations.'

Ron Bracey, clinical psychologist

'Those who love deeply never grow old; they may die of old age, but they die young.'

Benjamin Franklin

It's your funeral!

Imagining your own funeral is a good way of clarifying your own goals and values. Picture the scene in your mind and ask yourself: What do I want people to be saying about me when I'm gone? What do I want my life to have stood for?

'It's about good clean living, always being employed and having a happy family life.'

Stanley Wilkins, 86

Affirmative action

Affirmations are positive statements of intent in the present tense, which with repeated use can be used to improve positive thinking. For longevity, affirmation expert Jane Ducan suggests a sentence such as 'I am ageing with grace, gratitude and love for who I am' or 'I welcome the delights of ageing'. Repeat over and over - in your head or on paper - whenever negative thoughts start creeping in.

Only accept...

'Most centenarians do seem to have learned to deal with life on its own terms, to accept the loss of loved ones, and to continue to live with a certain amount of optimism.'

Jo Ann Warden, Florida Geriatric Research Program

'Whether you think you can or think you cannot, you are right.'

Henry Ford

'I'm interested in people. Getting involved with others, for instance, visiting sick and elderly friends - helps me through my own bad patches. And I couldn't possibly manage without prayer.'

Josephine Parkinson, 80

Frozen peace

If you fancy trying for immortality by having your body frozen, be careful who you choose to help. In 1975, a cryogenics company had to pay out US$1million compensation when it failed to pay its fuel bills - causing its frozen charges to thaw out...

Wise words

'Every day, make a couple of small changes that will make you feel better instantly. You'll find life gets easier very, very quickly.'

Richard Carlson, best-selling author

'The pessimist sees difficulty in every opportunity, the optimist sees opportunity in every difficulty.'

Winston Churchill

The Seven Ages of Man

Up until 7, you wish for puppies, shiny
bicycles and friends who stay for tea.
At ten you wish you were 18;
at 30, you wish you were 18;
at 40, you wish you were 30;
at 50, you wish you were 40;
at 60 you just wish for time again.
And at 90, you're either dead from all
the wishing, or you're one of the clever
people who never grew up.

© Ian the Poet

'*La joie de vivre est un devoir*'
Anonymous